conclusion

- Improved understanding of the critical phases of embryonic development and the capacity to identify these phases are of capital importance for diagnosing the period in which mortality occurs. Embryological diagnosis should be common practice and should be carried out on a daily basis. The two most sensitive phases during incubation are the start of blood circulation (first week) and the start of pulmonary respiration (last 5 days). This allows investigation of which parameter is incorrect (atmospheric composition, temperature, moisture, tilting, etc.), with a view to finding a solution to the problem.

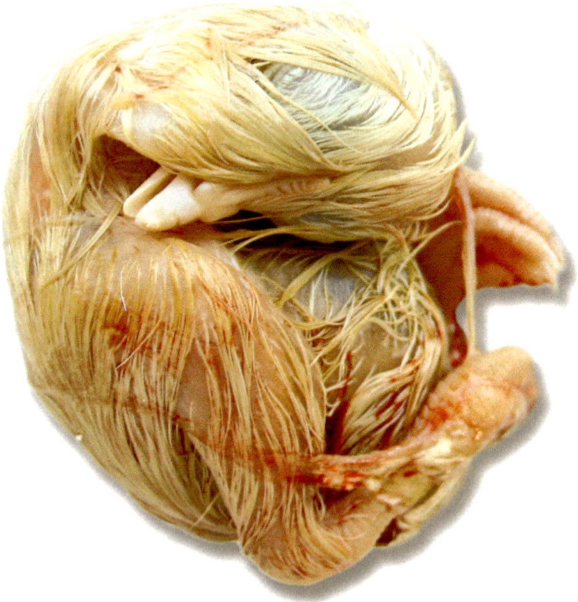

Day 21

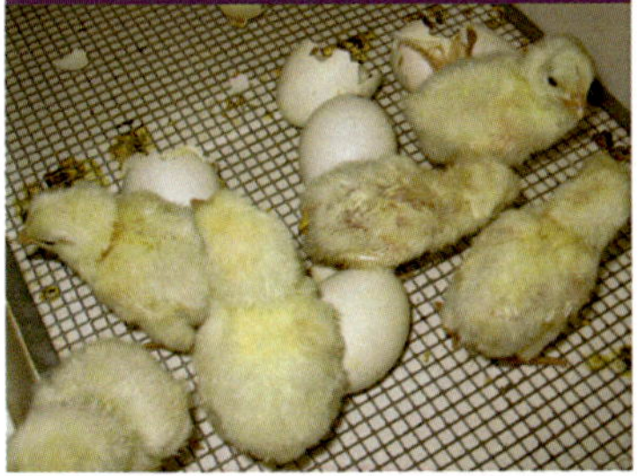

Day 21

- The chick uses its wing as a guide and its legs to turn on itself, and breaks through the shell in a circular manner using the "diamond". This begins about 12 hours after the start of pulmonary respiration, and causes an important increase in oxygen consumption. Pulmonary respiration is triggered by the high carbon dioxide concentration in the air chamber.

- Eclosion proper takes place 12-18 hours after the start of pecking, once the chick has been able to break 70-80 % of the shell. The chick emerges by itself from the shell and before resting to allow the down to dry.

- **The place where the shell has been pecked may indicate whether relative humidity was adequate (in the upper third of the egg), excessive (very close to the thick pole) or insufficient (near the equator of the egg). Difficulty breaking the shell, due to low humidity or insufficient ventilation, may prevent eclosion and cause embryo death from exhaustion.**

Day 20

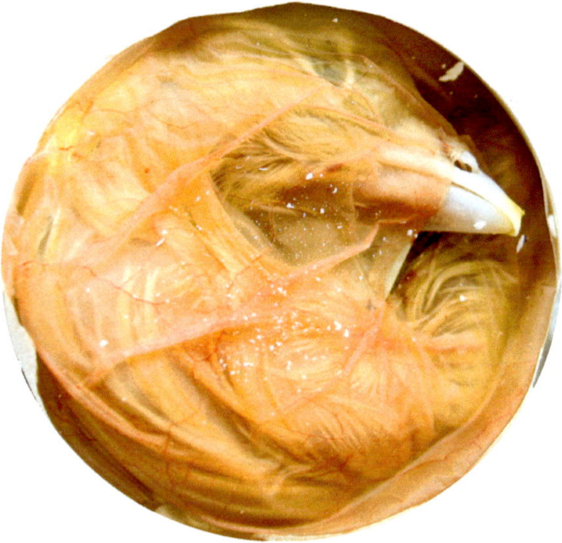

Day 20

- The embryo is now fully developed, weighs about 30 g and occupies the entire egg. The vitelline sac (30 % of its original size) is located within the abdominal cavity, with the still unhealed navel. This yolk is used by the chick as a source of food during the first 36 hours of life.

- About half-way through this day, pulmonary breathing becomes fully implemented, vocalization starts, and at the same time blood flow in the allantois decreases, and the latter starts to dry up. If the moisture or humidity in the incubator has been correct, the egg will have lost approximately 12 % of its initial weight.

- The chick perforates the internal membrane of the shell and breathes in the air chamber – gas exchange taking place through the pores of the shell. This is the point of eclosion, and the chick begins to break through the shell. Shell rupture is carried out using the beak, which is temporarily equipped with a small and hard prominence known as the "diamond".

Day 19

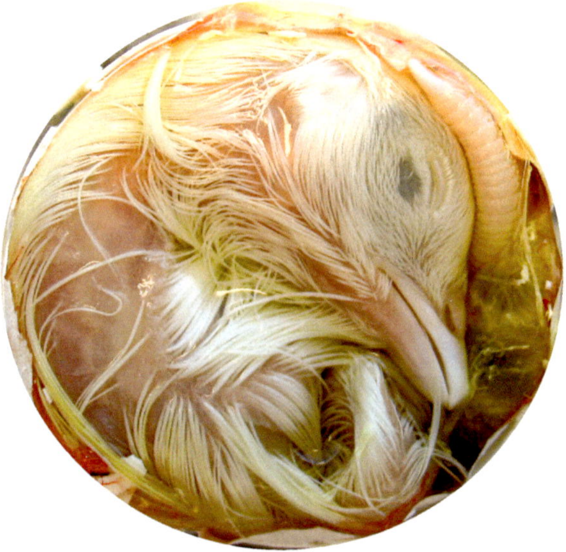

Day 19

- The embryo now weighs about 26 g and occupies the entire egg space except the air chamber. The head of the embryo is positioned below the right wing, and the beak points toward the air cell ready to perforate it.

- Yolk absorption accelerates and the amniotic fluid disappears.

- **On this day a large proportion of the chicks peck the air chamber, starting the transformation from gas exchange via the chorioallantoic membrane to gas exchange through the lungs. This change is gradual and is completed once histological lung development has concluded at the time when the chick begins to peck the egg shell (day 20-21) and thus needs a larger supply of oxygen due to the physical effort required. On days 18 and 19 mortality is often due to poorly positioned embryos.**

Day 18

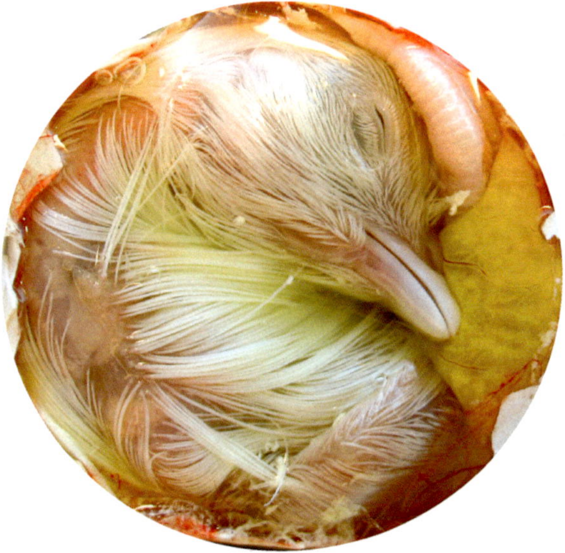

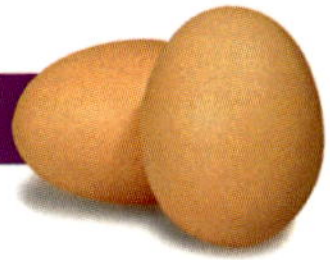

Day 18

- The yolk or vitellus begins to penetrate the abdominal cavity, and the amount of amniotic fluid decreases.

- This is the time (18-19 days) to transfer the eggs from the incubator to the hatching units to allow the embryo greater freedom of movement at hatching. Moreover, in this way hatching takes place in a tray, not in the inclined incubator setter trays. This step can be used to screen for clear and aborted eggs, and to perform in ovo vaccination. Following these actions, the trays are placed in the hatching units.

- From this day onwards intestinal development and function increase, as does the thermoregulatory capacity of the embryo. Correct ventilation, moisture and temperature in the hatching units are essential for hatching of the eggs. In this phase the maximum ventilation needs are reached (currently 33.4 m^3/hour for every 1000 eggs).

Day 17

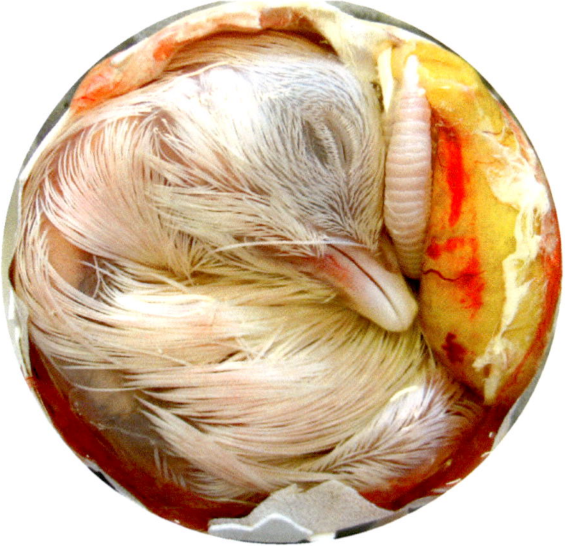

Day 17

- The head of the embryo is moving upwards from its original position, between the legs. Finally, the head should be located below the right wing, with its beak pointing towards the air chamber.
- The egg white has been completely reabsorbed, and the renal system of the embryo produces urates.
- **From this day onwards, embryo mortality increases, and up until the time of eclosion may represent two-thirds of the overall mortality. This situation worsens if the environmental conditions are not adequate, particularly as refers to ventilation flow, and also in the case of excessively porous eggs with high gas conductance (much more common in old hens).**

Day 16

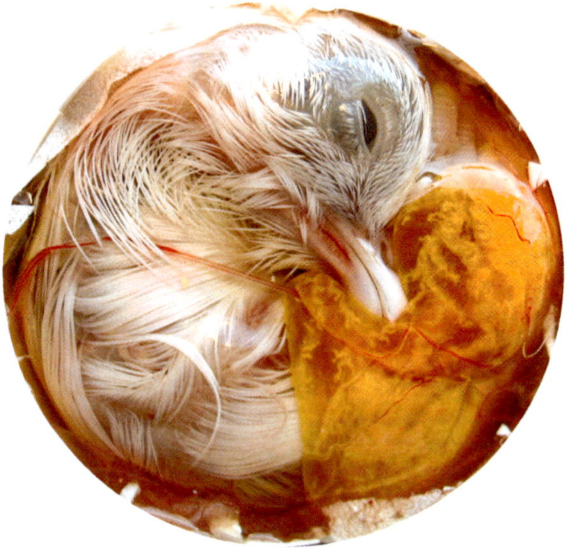

Day 16

- The embryo is completely covered in down. Nails and beak harden.
- The air chamber becomes quite large, and the embryo – which now weighs about 15 g – is positioned parallel to the long axis of the egg, with the head oriented towards the right, in preparation of eclosion.
- **The egg white has now disappeared, and absorption of the yolk begins. If the yolk presents clotting due to excessively high temperatures at the start of incubation (day 5), the embryo may die because it is unable to make use of the yolk.**
- The shell temperature increases, and in the last few days usually exceeds that of the incubator environment by about 2 °C.

Day 15

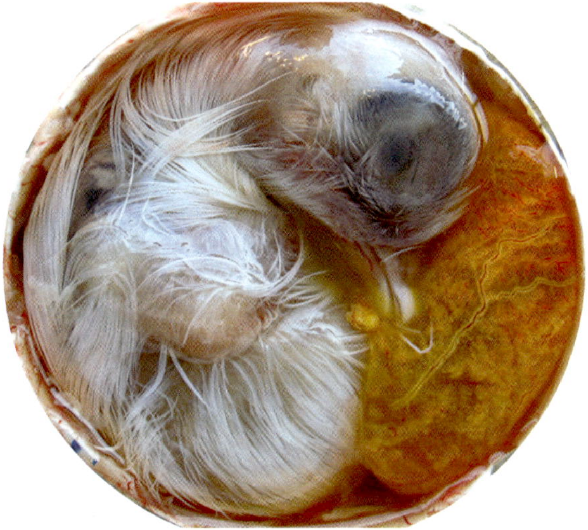

Day 15

- Few morphological changes are noted: the embryo and down continue to grow. The embryonic kidney becomes functional.

- The small intestine penetrates inside the body. Intestinal digestion and absorption begin at around day 15-16. In this way the embryo uses part of the proteins of the egg white once they have reached the amniotic fluid. The allantoic sac begins to accumulate excretions from the embryonic kidney, located to the left of the embryo.

- **The reduction in vitelline component accelerates and the albumen has almost completely disappeared. Egg white observed in embryos older than 15 days is indicative of a high average moisture content in the incubator, or a low average temperature, or both.**

Day 14

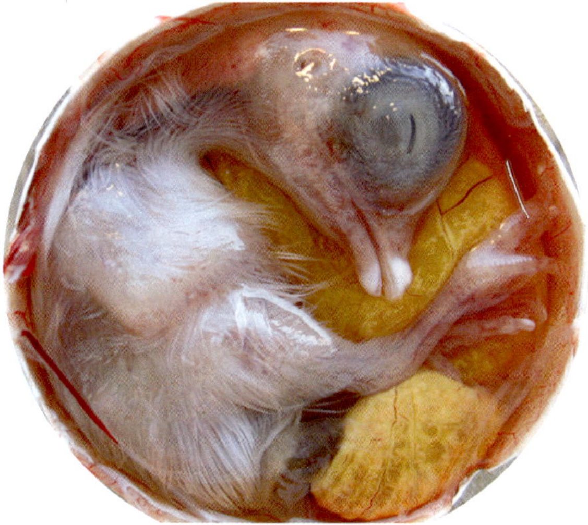

Day 14

- The down now almost covers the entire body and grows quickly. The eye is now closed.
- The embryo begins to rotate and gradually becomes positioned parallel to the long axis of the egg, turning the head towards the obtuse pole.
- The weight has now reached 9 g and the ventilation needs to be successively increased.

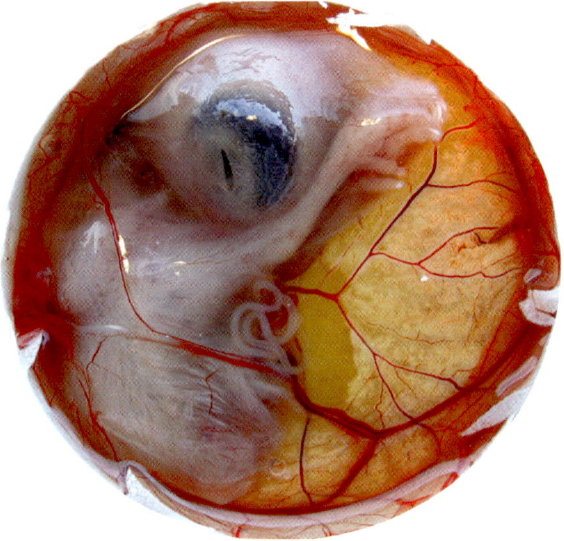

Day 13

1. Nail
2. Down growth

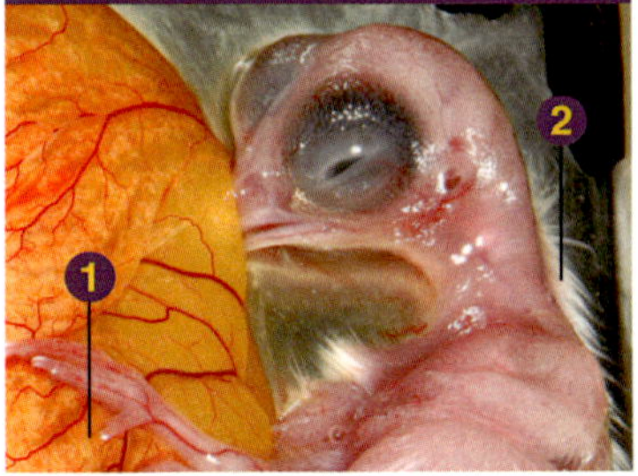

Day 13

- Important down growth. The eye is almost completely closed. Nails and scales appear.
- The allantois decreases in size and transforms into the chorioallantoic membrane.
- From this day onwards the embryo uses the proteins of the egg white, since opening of the seroamniotic communication allows the remaining albumen to penetrate the amniotic cavity. There is also a marked increase in calcium mobilization from the egg shell.

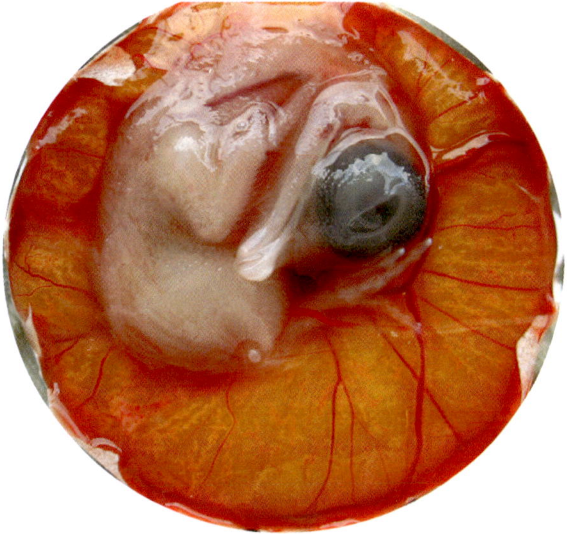

Day 12

1. Diamond
2. Upper eyelid
3. Lower eyelid

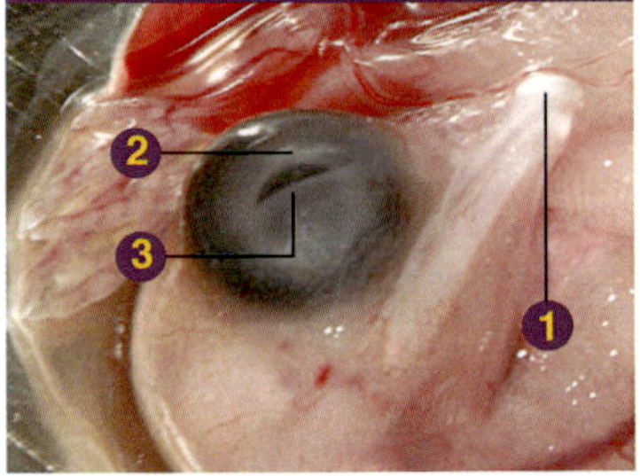

Day 12

- The eyelids are semi-joined at the edges; the lower eyelid covers two-thirds or even three-quarters of the cornea. The feather follicles cover the upper eyelid and surround the external auditory orifice.

- The digits of the feet are completely formed. Nails and beak acquire consistency, and the "diamond" is clearly visible.

- The embryo now weighs about 5 g. From this point onwards its proportional growth rate decreases, though in absolute terms it increases 2-4 g/day until transfer to the hatching unit. There is increased metabolic production of heat, and the need to eliminate it.

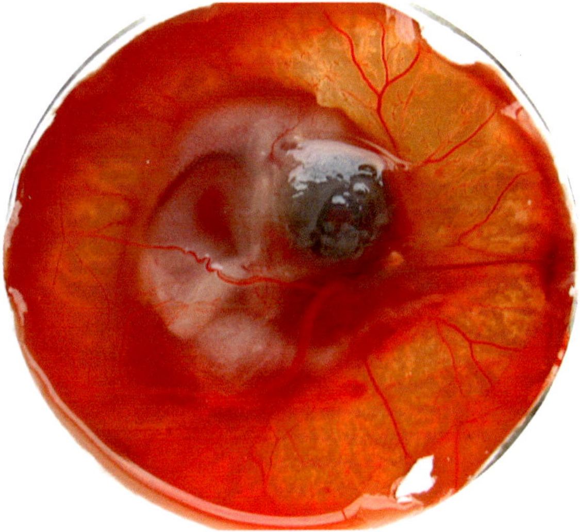

Day 11

1 Hair follicles

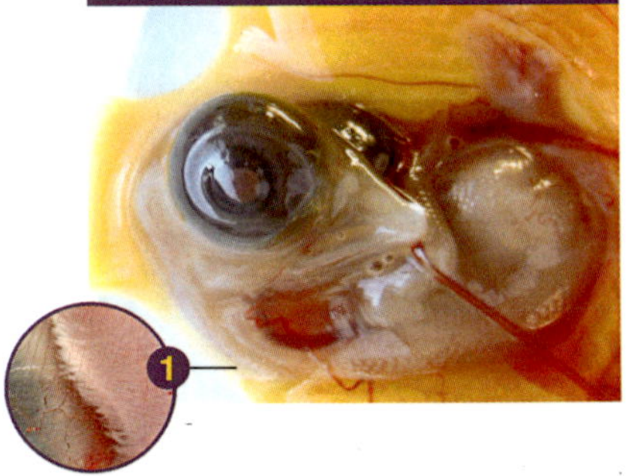

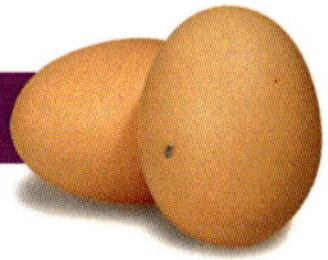

Day 11

- The embryo now looks like a chicken. Eyelid opening is elliptic in shape and tends to narrow.
- At the point the allantois is fully developed (internally lining the entire egg shell) and functional, while the vitelline component begins to decrease.
- **The feathers begin to appear. The embryos that die in this phase do not fill the egg, and the feathers show the time of death to have been between days 11 and 17. In addition, the head tends to be in the narrow or acute pole of the egg, and the egg contents appear brownish-red in color, typical of dry blood.**

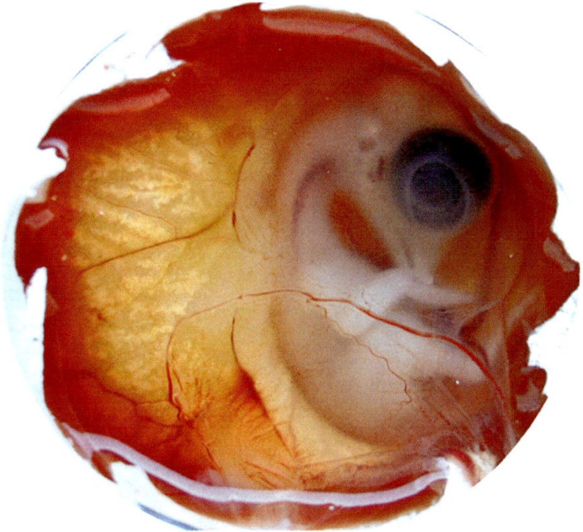

Day 10

1. Allantois
2. Vitelline sac
3. Vitelline membrane

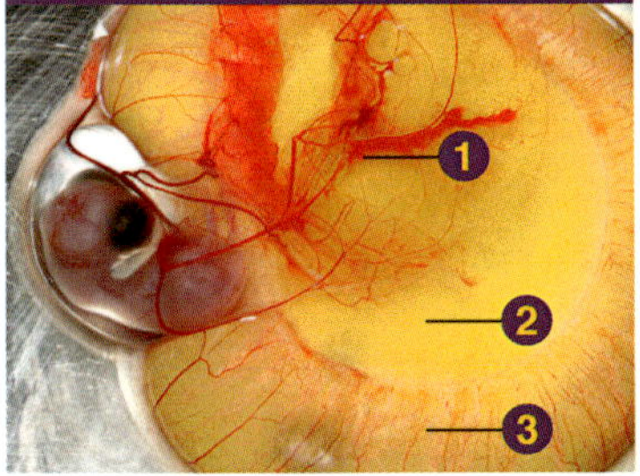

Day 10

- Extension of the distal portion of the extremities, the lower parts of which are now covered with feather follicles. Clearly visible "diamond"-shaped beak, and nostrils present as narrow openings.
- Growth of the eyelids, which begin to close.
- The vitelline membrane covers the entire yolk. The embryo is now more separated from the vitelline sac and is seen to float freely within the amniotic fluid. The weight of the embryo now reaches 2.5 g and the growth rate from this point onwards exceeds 100 % daily.

Day 9

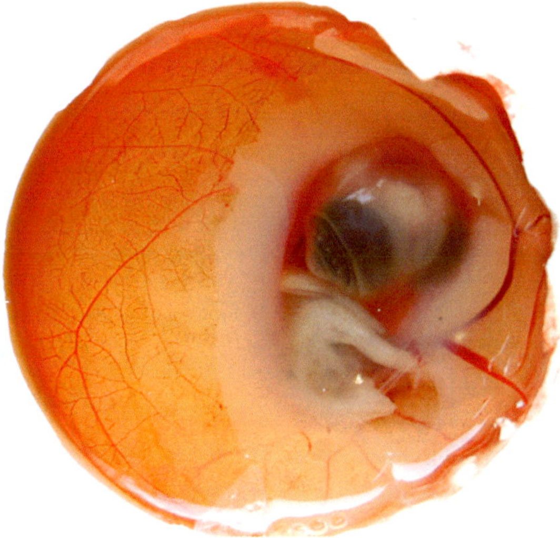

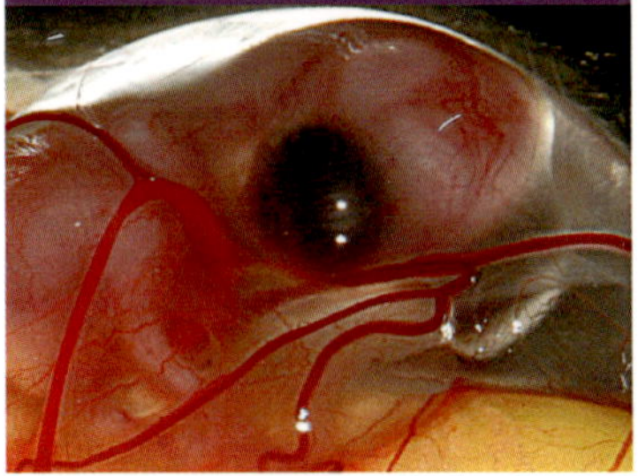

Day 9

- The nails appear, and the beak is able to open. Clearly differentiated limbs. The first feather follicles appear.
- Growth of the allantois and increased vitelline vascularization. The vitelline sac now fully envelops the yolk, and thus nutrient absorption intensifies.
- From this point onwards heat production on the part of the embryo increases, and the shell temperature is similar to that of the surrounding air. Tolerance to carbon dioxide continues to increase, though now the oxygen demands rise significantly and continuously.

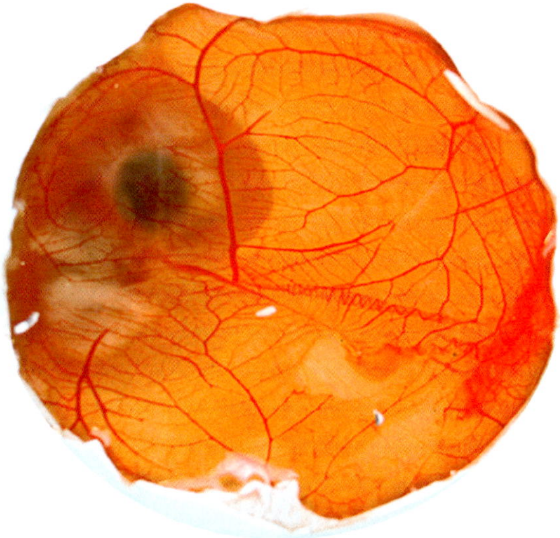

Day 8

1. Beak
2. External auditory canal
3. Amniotic sac

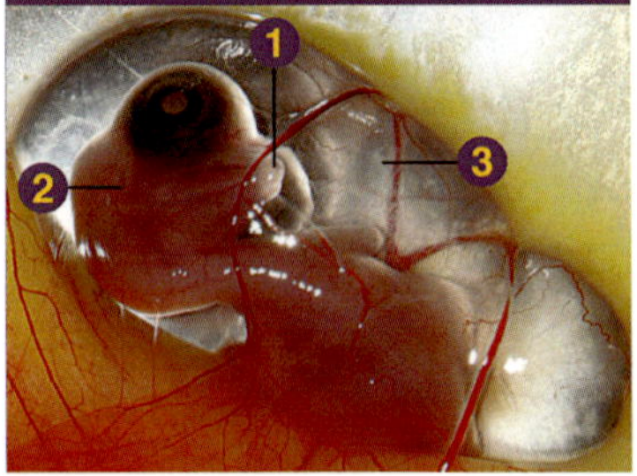

Day 8

- The vitelline membrane almost covers the entire yolk. Pigmentation of the eye is clearly visible. The upper and lower components of the beak are observable, as well as the wings and feet. The neck lengthens and the brain is almost fully housed within its cavity. Aperture of the external auditory canal visible.

- From this moment on, the phosphorus content of the phosphoproteins is used by the embryo for skeletal formation.

- **In this phase poor positioning of the embryo is sometimes seen, with the tarsus pointing towards the obtuse pole of the egg, visible beneath the air chamber. This may be because the egg has been placed in reverse, or the tilting angle of the incubator may be too small.**

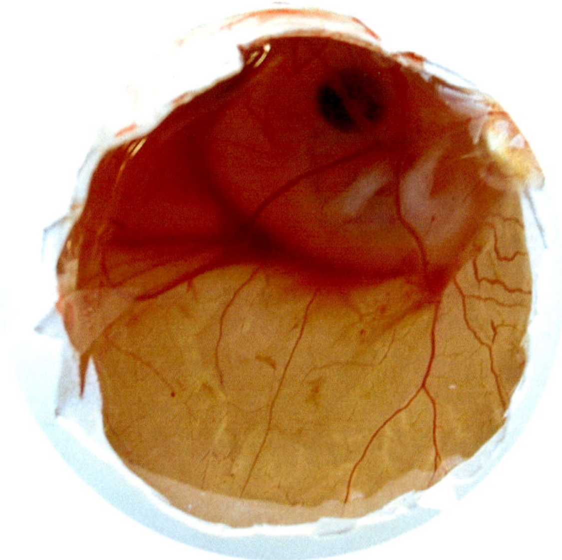

Day 7

1. Amniotic sac
2. Umbilical cord

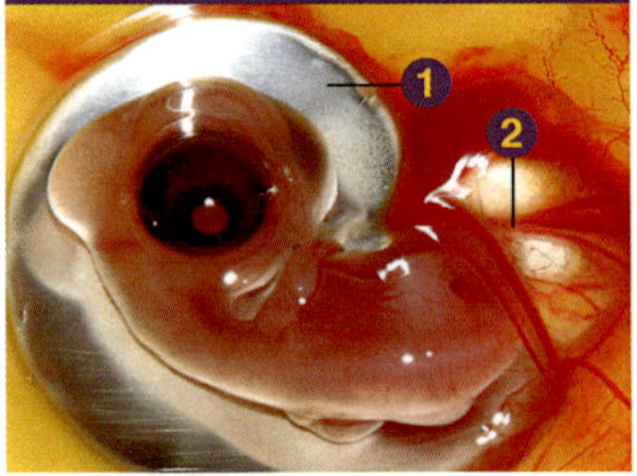

Day 7

- Narrowing of the neck, which now clearly separates head from trunk. The brain progressively penetrates the cephalic region; little by little its growth becomes proportionately smaller than the overall increase in embryo size. Formation of the beak.
- The embryo is still positioned over the surface of the vitelline sac, from which it is separated but in close contact. The embryo begins to adopt a bird-like shape: wings, legs and beak are clearly visible.
- From this moment on, the growth of the embryo (which now weighs 0.5 g) accelerates spectacularly.

Day 6

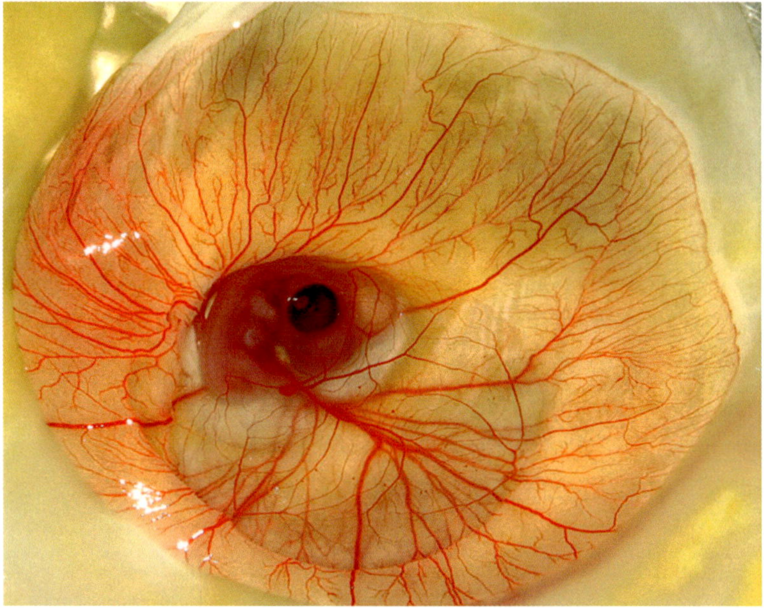

1 Amniotic cavity
2 Allantois

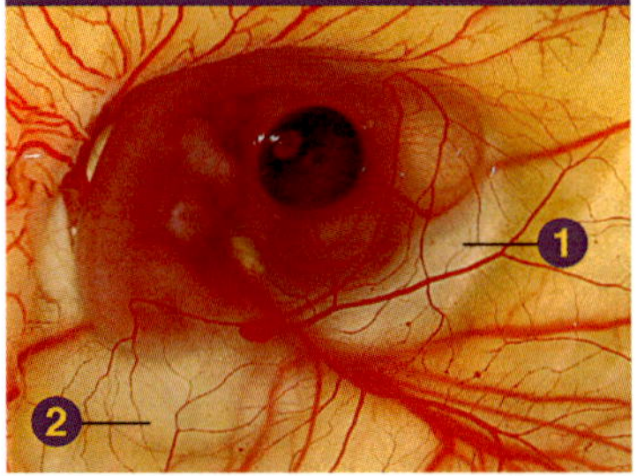

Day 6

- The vitelline membrane continues to grow and now surrounds more than half of the yolk. The first, second and third digits of the upper extremities separate, in the same way as the second and third digits of the lower extremities. The second digit is longer than the rest.

- The amniotic component decreases in size, thus making the embryo more sensitive to impacts during this period. Voluntary movements begin. The proventriculus and gizzard are already formed, and the liver begins to differentiate.

- At this point and until day 9, the oxygen demand and production of heat on the part of the embryo are very limited, and the generated heat is insufficient in itself to reach the body temperature of 37.5 °C. The shell temperature is usually 0.1 °C lower than the air in the incubator.

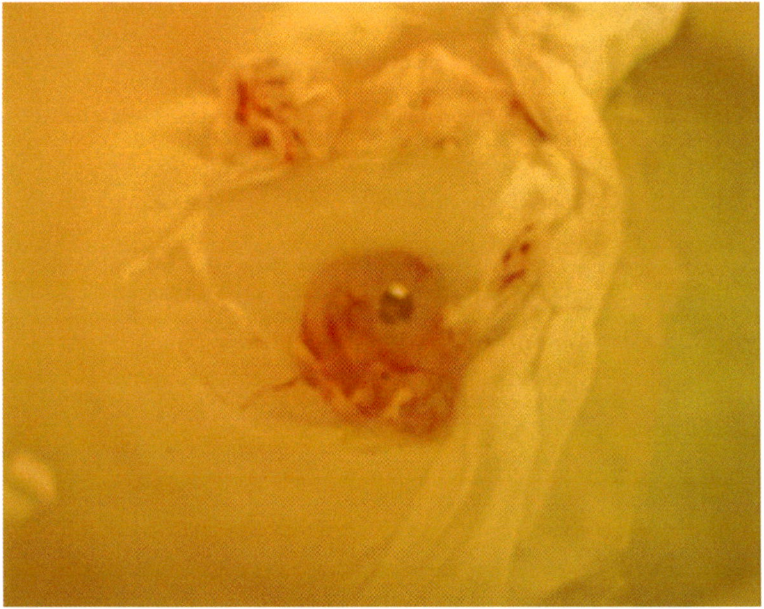

Day 5

1. Head extremity
2. Eye
3. Lower extremities
4. Upper extremities

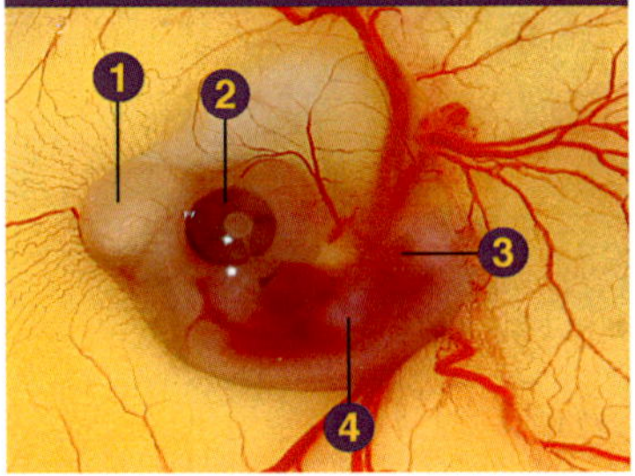

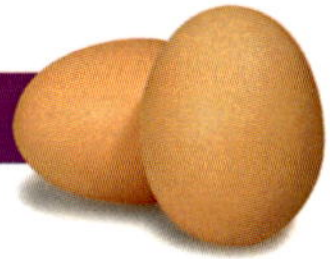

Day 5

- Appreciable increase in embryo size, with the adoption of a C-form shape; the head approaches the tail. Extension of the extremities, with differentiation of the digits on the hind limbs.

- The yolk is now very fluid; the presence of clots would indicate that the embryo has been exposed to excessively high temperatures at the start of incubation. In the first 5 days, two-thirds of the egg white water contents are used, resulting in a reduction in egg white volume, which becomes concentrated at the acute pole of the egg.

- **Eye pigmentation allows identification of mortality occurring between days 5 and 10 of incubation (normally very low; < 5 % of the total). An increase is usually attributable to bacterial contamination secondary to deficient nesting hygiene, inadequate egg disinfection or the condensation caused by sudden changes in temperature during preservation.**

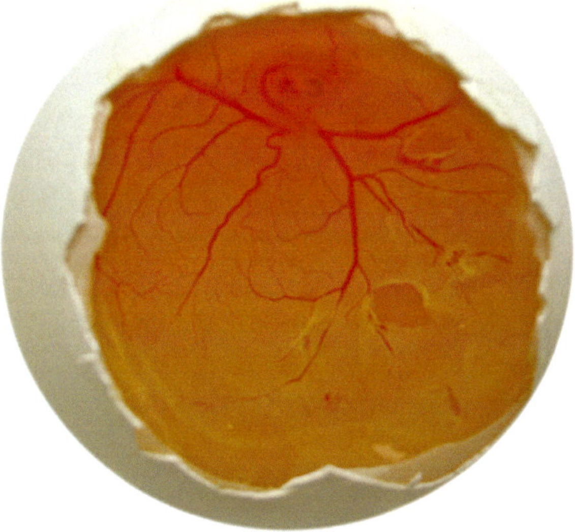

Day 4

1. Outline of the upper limb
2. Allantoic sac
3. Outline of the hind limb
4. Ocular globe

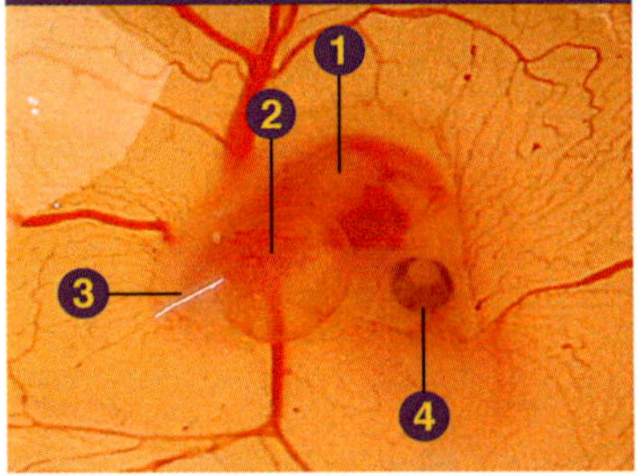

Day 4

- Development of the amniotic cavity, which surrounds the embryo and is filled with amniotic fluid that protects the embryo and allows it mobility. The allantoic sac appears: this structure plays an important role in respiration, calcium absorption and waste storage.

- The chorioallantois, which results from the fusion of both membranes, is connected to the shell membrane. This is the respiratory organ of the embryo up until day 18-19. The blood that circulates through its vessels is oxygenated by the air that penetrates through the pores of the shell, helps eliminate carbon dioxide towards the exterior, and transports oligoelements and minerals – fundamentally calcium from the shell.

- The embryo begins to metabolize vitelline lipids and proteins, giving rise to an increase in ammonia, carbon dioxide and lactic acid – substances that may cause death due to intoxication if not quickly and effectively eliminated by the newly formed capillary vessels.

Day 3

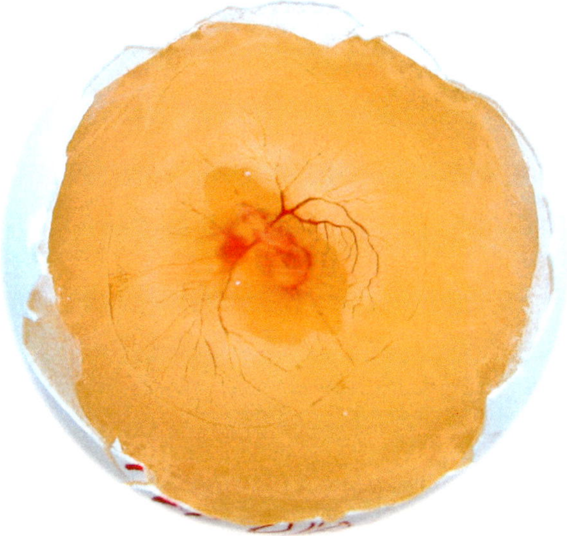

1. Posterior portion
2. Neural tube
3. Formation of the heart
4. Outline of the head

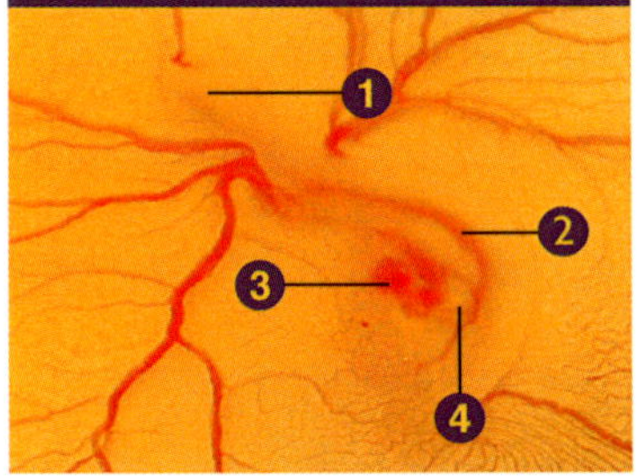

Day 3

- The embryo rests on its left side. The trunk, head and brain can be distinguished. The vitelline membrane extends over the surface of the yolk. The heart structures are already visible and begin to beat, and blood circulation starts.

- **From two and a half to four days, dead embryos are distinguished by the presence of a ring of blood. Excessively high temperatures between days one and three cause brain ectopia.**

- Up until day three, the enzyme resources of the embryo are too limited to degrade complex molecules; as a result, mostly simple substances in free state are used, such as glucose from the egg white and amino acids from the yolk.

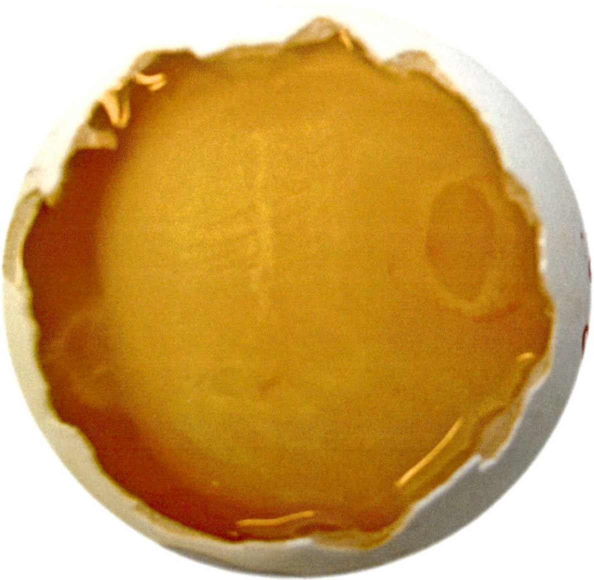

Day 2

1. Embryo
2. Extraembryonic appendage

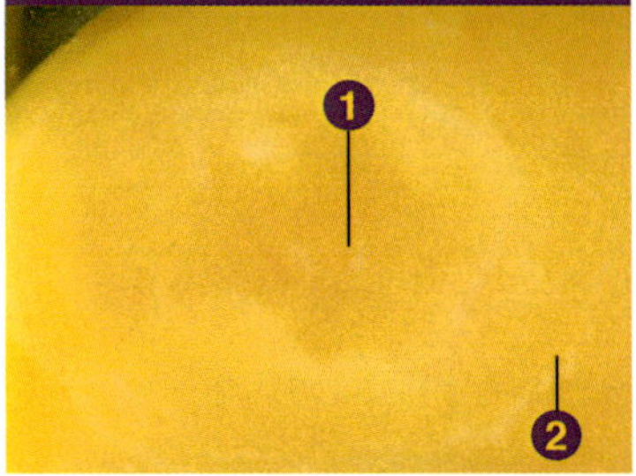

Day 2

- The first groove or sulcus appears at the center of the blastoderm. The extraembryonic appendages give rise to the vitelline membrane, which will play an important role in nutrition of the embryo.

- **In the first two days the embryo is very sensitive, due to the fragility of the blastoderm and the formation of the vascular network (towards 40 hours of life), and is also much more susceptible to excess carbon dioxide.**

- Mortality in this stage is evidenced by a cream color of the vitelline membrane, with a diameter of between 5-20 mm, and in which the blood vessels are not yet visible. The causes of mortality are diverse: prolonged storage or storage under inadequate conditions, incorrect disinfection of the eggs, or too high a temperature at the start of incubation.

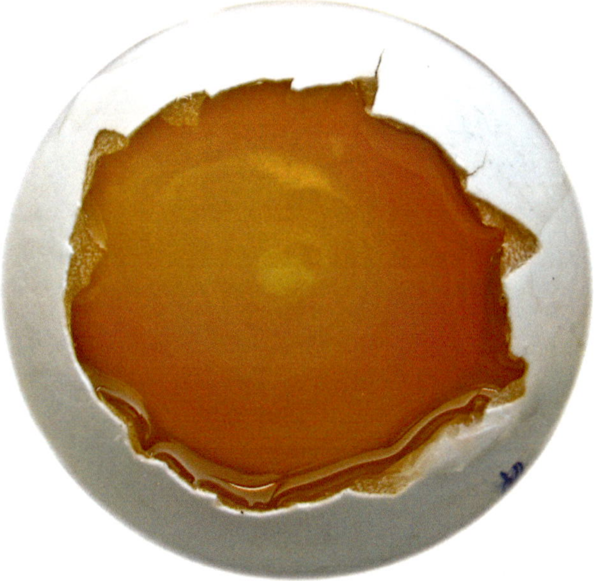

Day 1

1. Pellucid zone
2. Opaque zone

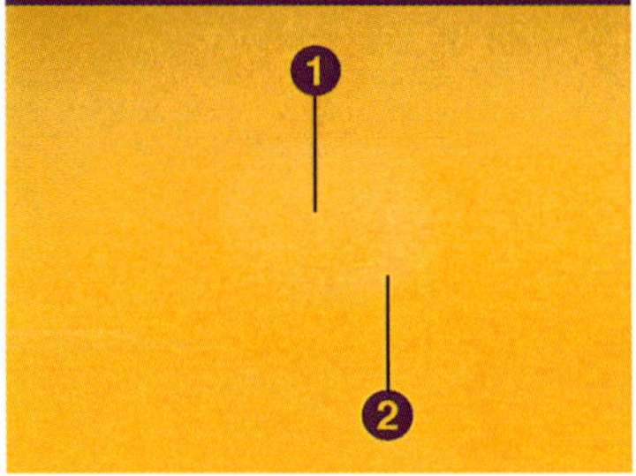

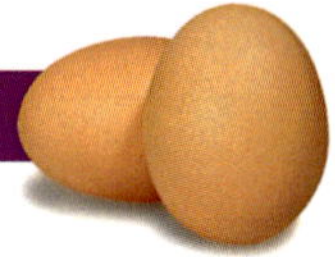

Day 1

- The germinal disc is in the blastoderm stage. The segmentation cavity, under the zona pellucida, appears as a dark ring. Within the first 24 hours the digestive system, spine and nervous system begin to develop.
- With development of the blastoderm on the surface of the yolk a membrane also begins to develop that later on will fully envelop the yolk: the vitelline sac.
- In aborted eggs, even in the first hours of incubation, we always observe yolk adherence to the egg white, along with a series of embryonic development bands over the yolk. In contrast, in an infertile egg, only a germinal vesicle is observed.

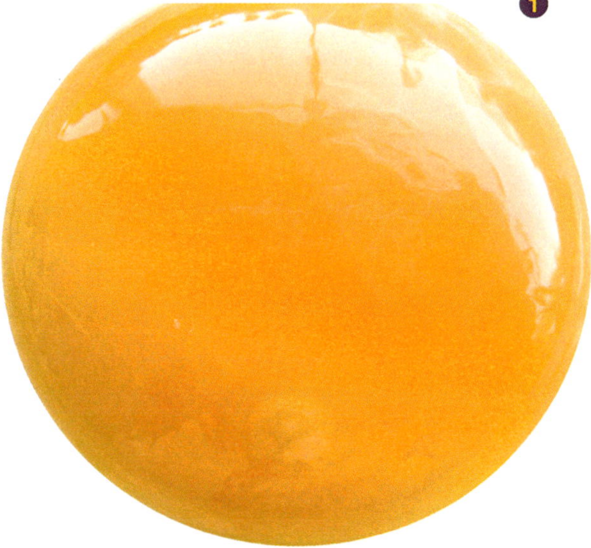

Day 0

1 Fertile

2 Infertile

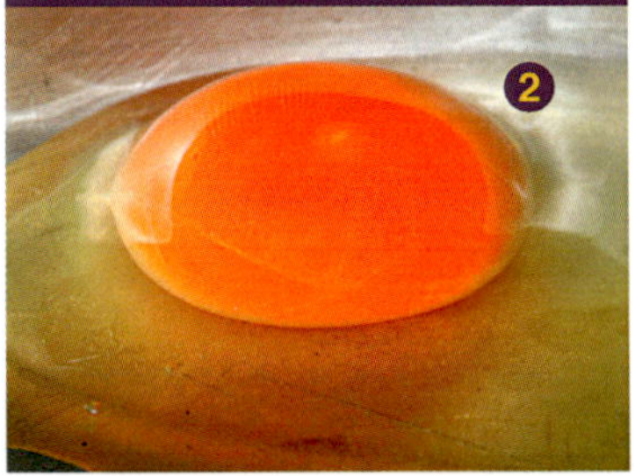

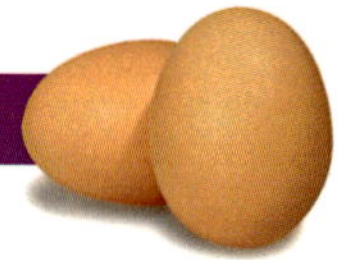

Day 0

- **Infertile**
  The embryonic disc of a sterile egg presents accumulated white material at its center.

- **Fertile**
  The fertilized embryonic disc looks like a ring: it has a brighter central zone where the embryo is located.

- **The embryo has now been developing for over 24 hours in the oviduct of the hen. When the egg reaches a temperature of under 22 °C, it remains in a latent life stage. Such cooling must be gradual in order to prevent an increase in early embryonic mortality.**

- In situations of breeder hen stress, the embryonic disc is very small – this can cause problems for the resumption of development once the eggs are loaded in the incubator.

Authors

Dr. Ricardo Cepero Briz.
Department of Animal Production. Faculty of Veterinary Science.
University of Zaragoza (Spain).

Ricardo Marco García.
Veterinarian specialized in aviculture.

Warning:
Veterinary science is constantly evolving, as are pharmacology and the other sciences. Inevitably, it is therefore the responsibility of the veterinary clinician to determine and verify the dosage, the method of administration, the duration of treatment and any possible contraindications to the treatments given to each individual patient, based on his or her professional experience. Neither the publisher nor the author can be held liable for any damage or harm caused to people, animals or properties resulting from the correct or incorrect application of the information contained in this book.

This book has been published originally in spanish under the title:
Atlas de desarrollo embrionario

ISBN spanish edition: 978-84-940402-6-9

For this english edition:

Plaza Antonio Beltrán Martínez n° 1, planta 8 - letra I
(Centro empresarial El Trovador)
50002 Zaragoza - Spain

Translation:
Grupo Asís Biomedia, S.L.

Design and layout:
Servet editorial - Grupo Asís Biomedia, S.L.
www.grupoasis.com
info@grupoasis.com

ISBN: 978-84-942449-8-8
D.L.: Z 787-2014

Printed in Spain

ATLAS OF EMBRYONIC DEVELOPMENT

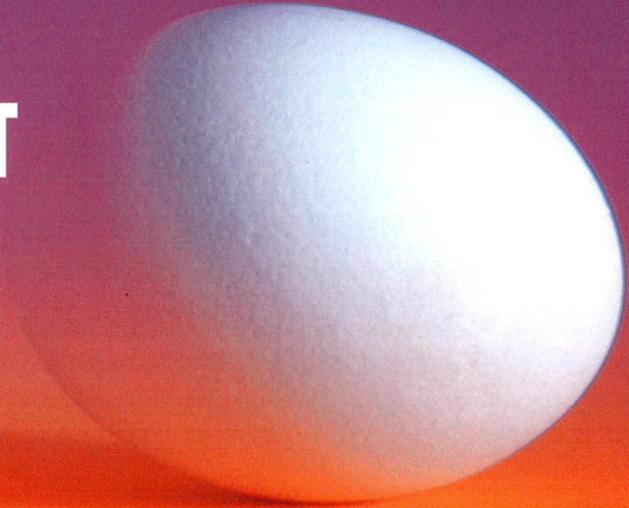

SERVET